# YOUR KNOWLEDGE HAS VALUE

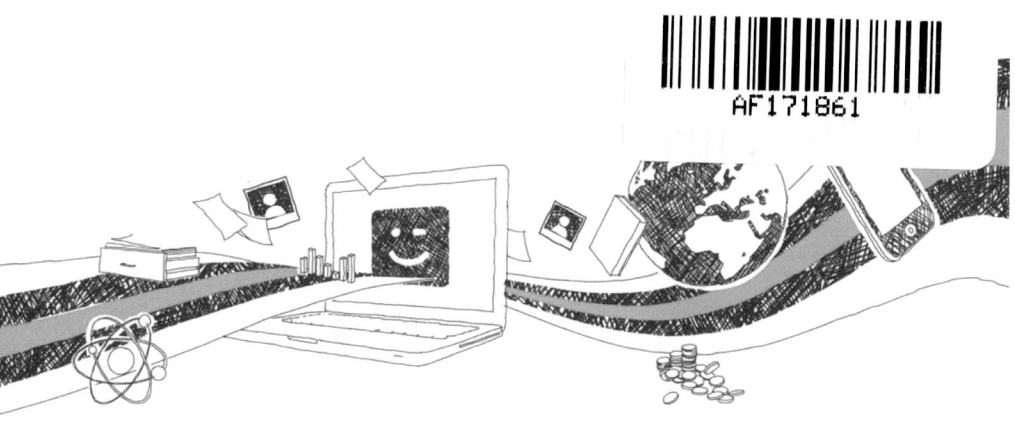

- We will publish your bachelor's and master's thesis, essays and papers

- Your own eBook and book - sold worldwide in all relevant shops

- Earn money with each sale

Upload your text at www.GRIN.com and publish for free

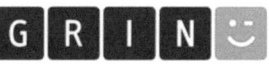

**Bibliographic information published by the German National Library:**

The German National Library lists this publication in the National Bibliography; detailed bibliographic data are available on the Internet at http://dnb.dnb.de .

This book is copyright material and must not be copied, reproduced, transferred, distributed, leased, licensed or publicly performed or used in any way except as specifically permitted in writing by the publishers, as allowed under the terms and conditions under which it was purchased or as strictly permitted by applicable copyright law. Any unauthorized distribution or use of this text may be a direct infringement of the author s and publisher s rights and those responsible may be liable in law accordingly.

**Imprint:**

Copyright © 2018 GRIN Verlag
Print and binding: Books on Demand GmbH, Norderstedt Germany
ISBN: 9783668723016

**This book at GRIN:**

https://www.grin.com/document/428646

Leonard Kahungu

# Contemporary Themes In Health Care. Incidence And Management Of Coronary Heart Disease In The United Kingdom

GRIN Verlag

**GRIN - Your knowledge has value**

Since its foundation in 1998, GRIN has specialized in publishing academic texts by students, college teachers and other academics as e-book and printed book. The website www.grin.com is an ideal platform for presenting term papers, final papers, scientific essays, dissertations and specialist books.

**Visit us on the internet:**

http://www.grin.com/

http://www.facebook.com/grincom

http://www.twitter.com/grin_com

CONTEMPORARY THEMES IN HEALTH CARE: INCIDENCE AND MANAGEMENT OF CORONARY HEART DISEASE IN THE UNITED KINGDOM

**Introduction**

According to the World Health Organisation (WHO), cardiovascular diseases (CVD) are the leading cause of premature deaths in industrialized countries. WHO estimates that this number will reach more than twenty-three million people by the year 2030 (Williams et al., 2010). CVD are classified as lifestyle diseases since they are attributed to unhealthy behaviours in the human life. Typically, CVD is a collective term used to refer to a group of disorders with some common health determinants that are linked to atherosclerosis. Atherosclerosis is a condition that describes the stiffening of the artery walls (King et al., 2017). In the United Kingdom (UK), CVD affects about seven million people and has since been identified as the leading cause of disability and death. It is also established that CVD causes one in four premature deaths in the UK, in which it accounted for about 26% of deaths recorded in England in the year 2015. CVD has also been associated with escalating financial burdens in the UK healthcare system, in which the condition consumes over £9 billion annually, costing the UK economy over £19 billion each year (Bhatnagar et al., 2016). The annual economic cost estimates incorporate premature deaths, informal costs, and disabilities.

**Coronary Heart Disease**

Consequently, the coronary heart disease (CHD) is the most common type of CVD. CHD is described as the narrowing of the coronary arteries along with the blood vessels supplying blood and oxygen to the heart. It is also known as the coronary artery disease and occurs as a result of cholesterol accumulation on the artery walls. This narrows the arteries and reduces the flow of blood the heart. In some instances, the constriction of the arteries may cause a clot, which obstructs blood circulation in the heart muscles (Hollis et al., 2017). Coronary arteries are blood vessel networks found on the surface of the heart, and they function by nourishing the heart muscles. Thus, the resulting constriction due to increased cholesterol levels interferes with the normal functions of the heart, especially during physical activities. Initially, the reduction of blood supply remains asymptomatic until fatty acids build up in the coronary arteries, leading to significant symptomatic manifestations.

The existing literature indicates that CHD starts with damage or injuries along the inner walls of the coronary arteries. This causes fatty plagues to deposit and build up at the damaged wall. The deposited materials mainly consist of cholesterol along with cellular products, in which the accumulation is known as atherosclerosis. When the piece rapture, the platelets accumulate on the damaged site, in attempts to repair the blood vessel tissue. Leads to the formation of clumps, which increase the risk of blocking the coronary arteries, which reduce or prevent the blood flow to the heart (De Backer et al., 2013). This increases the risk of heart attack, which is one of the significant manifestations of CHD.

Just like CVD, CHD is classified as the leading cause of death in the UK as well as across the globe. Notably, it is estimated that CHD causes the death of one in seven men and also one in twelve women across the world. It also triggers the death of more than sixty-six thousand deaths in the UK, which translated to about 180 deaths on a daily basis or one fatality after every eight minutes. A heart attack causes most deaths in CHD. Additionally, over two million people in the UK are currently living with CHD. This indicates that CHD remains a major public health concern in the United Kingdom, and hence a contemporary theme in the healthcare system (Hollis et al., 2017). Thus, it is paramount to understand the incidence and the management of CHD in attempts to reduce the financial, human, and population costs associated with the prevalence of CHD in the UK.

**Risk Factors Influencing CHD Incidence**

Studies indicate that CHD is the primary cause of death among the South Asian population in the UK. This is because the risk of getting CHD is higher in the South Asian population compared to the indigenous white population. The risk is placed at 46% (in men) and 51% (in women), higher in the South Asian community living in the UK. Additionally, the South Asian community is 50% likely to die from CHD more than any other population in the UK. In other words, South Asian immigrants are 1.5% times more likely to die from CHD and other related morbidities (Danese et al., 2016). Unfortunately, this population has not also benefited from reduced CHD deaths in the last few decades as it is the case with other population groups in the UK. These observations are attributed to multifaceted socioeconomic and genetic factors characterising this population. For instance, it is estimated that the South Asian populations have high smoking levels and deprived socioeconomic status more than any other group living in the UK. Besides, most individuals from the South Asian population seek medical attention when CHD is at advanced levels, reducing the chances of survival (Bhatnagar et al., 2016). Low-income populations living in England are more prone to CHD as opposed to those living in areas with favourable socioeconomic factors. Moreover, people from black races are more likely to die from CHD compared to the white population.

Consequently, severe hypertension increases the risk of suffering from CHD by two times. The risk of getting CHD in pre-hypertension varies from one individual to another. Hypertension occurs due to elevated blood pressure and is caused by several metabolic disorders attributed to poor lifestyles such as diabetes. In particular, diabetes increases the risk of developing CVD by two to four times (King et al., 2017). Diabetes has also been associated with several CHD factors including obesity, dyslipidaemia, as well as hypertension. Nonetheless, the existing evidence shows that diabetes is a risk factor in itself. Glycated haemoglobin controls the blood pressure body mass index, along with blood lipids, which is also the primary component with influence diabetes incidences. This shows that diabetes may be considered as a risk factor in the CHD incidences. As previously observed in South Asian populations, smoking is one of the significant factors influencing CHD risks (King et al., 2017). Women who smoke are more likely to get CHD compared to men. The risk arising from smoking has been identified as the most modifiable factor in the management and prevention of CVD.

Obesity is linked to other CHD risk factors such as hypertension, diabetes, and dyslipidaemia, among others. Normally, adipose tissues release considerable bioactive mediators that alter metabolism activities, influencing insulin resistance and body mass accumulation, which are the primary type 2 diabetes precursor. These factors cause a number of health complications such as blood pressure, coagulation, and lipids alteration, causing atherosclerosis and endothelial dysfunction. Poor socioeconomic status in the UK significant factor influencing CHD occurrence (Williams et al., 2010). Trends in populations with favourable socioeconomic backgrounds in smoking, cholesterol, and blood pressure are consistent with reducing CHD mortalities, but obesity and diabetes occurrences in low-income families are contradicting some of these developments. Little has also been done to address healthcare disparities in the UK populations. Sedentary lifestyles coupled with poor diet increase the risk of CHD. This is attributed to the accumulation of calories, increasing the risk of metabolic disorders that trigger the onset of CHD and CVD mortalities (Hollis et al., 2017). It is estimated that adults who exercise fifteen minutes a day have a longer life expectancy rate and reduce the risk of major lifestyle morbidities and mortalities. Thus, this indicates that physical activities reduce the risk of CHD. Physical exercises reduce the muscle tension, which improves the blood flow throughout the body.

**Contemporary CHD Management**

Notably, CHD is a chronic condition that develops throughout the lifespan of an individual and symptoms are likely to manifest themselves at advanced stages. Although mortality incidences caused by the coronary artery disease has reduced in the recent past, it remains the leading cause of premature deaths in the United Kingdom (Bhatnagar et al., 2016). Preventing CHD incidents remains a considerable public health challenge for policymakers, general population, and healthcare stakeholders in the UK and the world. A review of CHD risk factors strongly shows that this condition is connected to lifestyle, particularly sedentary lifestyles, psychosocial stress, unhealthy dietary plans, and the use of tobacco products among other factors. Thus, CHD prevention and management necessitates the involvement of the concerned stakeholders at an individual, community, and institutional levels in the eradication, or minimisation of the effects of CHD and associated health complications (Williams et al., 2010). The management of CHD is guided by the contemporary cardiovascular epidemiological knowledge and evidence-based clinical practices.

Although there are some genetic and inherent factors associated with CHD susceptibility, coronary heart disease along with other cardiovascular diseases are largely linked to lifestyle behaviours. Thus, most of the recommendations are based on behaviour management, which has to be strengthened by effective and robust policies in the United Kingdom. Therefore, the control and prevention of CHD starts during the gestation period and continues to the end of life (Danese et al., 2016). This indicates that preventive, management and interventions addressing CHD target all stages in the human lifespan, with a particular focus on the middle-aged and senior citizens with established cardiovascular conditions. Individuals categorised as high-risk populations with regards to cardiovascular events are also the primary target in preventive and management strategies (Williams et al., 2010). High-risk populations include men and women with high blood pressure, smoking habits, obesity, diabetes and other health complications. Two main CVD and CHD management and prevention approaches are either categorised as population strategy or the high-risk strategy.

The population strategy targets a reduction of CHD incidence rates at the community level by addressing behaviour and environmental modification. These changes often target the population at large, in this case, the Britons. This strategy is largely based on public and community health policies as well as interventions (De Backer et al., 2013). The population strategy benefits the community but has fewer benefits to specific individuals. On the other hand, the high-risk strategy aims at reducing CVD on population groups associated with the highest risk. High-risk programmes significantly benefit the society at an individual level but remain ineffective at the community level. Over the past years, population strategy has been identified as the most effective and cost-efficient approach for managing CVD (Hollis et al., 2017). Nonetheless, the efficiency of high strategy programmes has improved in the recent past with the introduction of tailored approaches targeting populations believed to be highly vulnerable to coronary artery disease.

Apparently, heighten. cardiovascular risk is increasingly becoming a lifelong issue, illustrating that various exposures even before birth may increase the risk of suffering from CVD. This illustrates the significance of lifestyle management, especially during the young age as it considerably lowers the CHD susceptibility. Ethical and legal complications complicate the development of advanced studies to establish the impact of lifestyle management in teenagers or young age. Nevertheless, universal studies indicate that earlier interventions are fundamental in reducing the risk of CHD as the age progresses (Hollis et al., 2017). For instance, smoking cessation at a very young age considerably reduces the risk of CHD at an advanced age. The management of CHD is paramount as it improves the quality of life and also reduces financial and cost burden associated with CHD and cardiovascular diseases in general.

**CHD Management Recommendations for Practice**

Evidently, the literature review identifies the South Asian group as the most vulnerable group in the UK population. Incidentally, the South Asian population is one of the marginalized groups in Britain (Prince et al., 2015). One of the reasons influencing high CHD incidence rates within the South Asian group is attributed to late diagnosis, lifestyle preferences, and socioeconomic issues. This indicates a strong correlation between healthcare disparities and the CHD incidence in this population. Whereas the rest of population groups, especially the Whites, have recorded a significant drop in mortalities caused by CHD, marginalised communities led by the South Asian group continue to witness increased patterns of deaths caused by coronary heart disease (Yusuf et al., 2016). As a consequence, it is paramount to consider the development of robust measures that can be used in reducing healthcare disparities affecting the marginalized communities. Healthcare disparities are the leading cause of healthcare inefficiencies in the UK. One of the best strategies for addressing healthcare disparities in the UK is by promoting cultural awareness in the healthcare industry (De Backer et al., 2013). Thus, the first commendation involves the promotion of cultural awareness in the UK healthcare systems, especially in regions with high marginalised populations.

The multicultural theories require healthcare practitioners to ensure they deliver culturally competent care. Evidence-based studies indicate that cultural competence plays a central role in addressing care disparities as it improves the relationship between the care practitioners and the marginalized communities (Tillin et al., 2014). This approach requires the healthcare fraternity to understand the cultural practices, values, and beliefs that can be used in enhancing the prevention of CHD. For instance, understanding the indigenous physical exercises can help healthcare practitioners and policymakers dealing with marginalised communities advocate the inclusion of cultural games that promote physical fitness in school programmes and community centres (Roth et al., 2015). The delivery of culturally competent healthcare improves the relationship between minority communities and healthcare community, enhancing the level of confidence of the minority groups in seeking the primary medical services. This commendation will be central in reducing the CHD incidence rates in the South Asian population, which is considered as the high-risk group in the UK (Hollis et al., 2017). The strategy ought to be replicated in other marginalized community considered at high risk of developing CHD, in efforts to standardize the gains made in the prevention and management of the major cardiovascular disease.

Apparently, CHD is significantly associated with various health conditions linked to lifestyle diseases such as diabetes, hypertension, obesity, and abnormal cholesterol levels. As a recommendation, the UK healthcare system should consider mounting rigorous and sustained awareness campaigns aimed at increasing the level of consciousness regarding the implications of unhealthy lifestyles (Prince et al., 2015). This approach is based on theoretical principles linked to the health belief model. This model is based on the assumptions that providing the target population with the risk associated with certain behaviours encourages them to stop the discouraged lifestyles. Furthermore, educating the public concerning the benefits of adopting healthy life practices is likely to promote adherence to good and healthy lifestyles (King et al., 2017). These approaches are fundamental in the promotion of healthy lifestyles in the UK population, especially by addressing sedentary lifestyles. This would reduce the incidence rates of various diseases that increase the risk of CHD, such as diabetes. It would also enhance the management of conditions that increase the risk of CHD, as a secondary prevention and management approach.

Another commendation related to public health promotion strategy concerns educating the public about the importance of regular medical check-ups. This will facilitate the management of the lipids, blood, glucose, and other risk factors. Improved management of various risk factors is fundamental, particularly in asymptomatic patients. The existing literature shows that CHD progression is virtually lifelong, where various body conditions contribute to the development of the coronary artery disease, especially in advanced age. This indicates that appropriate interventions mounted when a person is very young can reduce the vulnerability of getting heart diseases. Alternatively, screening for lipids, glucose, and other factors increase the risk of CVD should be integrated with the primary healthcare services. This is likely to enhance the ability to promote primary and secondary prevention as well as the management of CHD incidences in the UK population.

Particularly, lipid management should be based on a five-year cycle of measuring lipid profile, which has to start at the age of twenty years. This should be repeated annually when the patient's lipid profile shows some abnormalities or if the patient has been diagnosed with CHD. Consequently, glucose management has to be measured in a cycle of every three years starting at the age of 45 years. This management can also start at a very young age when the patient is considered at high risk of CHD or CVD (Daoud et al., 2014). Lastly, the blood pressure management should focus on BP measurement in every year. This can be done more often if there are clinical requirements. Coronary artery calcification (CAC) screening in asymptomatic patients, especially those with multislice cardiac CT is paramount in the management of CHD. CAC screening would focus on men between the age of 45 and 75 years and women between the age of 55-75 years. The CAC screening results must be used to guide therapeutic decisions and management interventions.

Evidently, the review indicates that evidence-based guidelines regarding CHD risks and the impact of appropriate management remains flimsy due to legal and ethical complications. This hinders the ability to develop lifelong management of CHD risks (Williams et al., 2010). The scanty details have already shown a significant link between lifestyle preferences in young people and the risk of developing CHD in their adult or old-age life. This is sufficient reason to warrant more intensified research targeting young populations in attempts to ensure CHD risks have been efficiently managed right from the childhood to advanced age (Osborn et al., 2015). Therefore, it is paramount for the healthcare fraternity to develop practical approaches that would address legal and ethical concerns and at the same time lead to the contribution of knowledge in efforts to enhance the contemporary evidence-based guidelines in the management of CHD. Besides, CHD and CVD have since been considered as the leading cause of premature deaths in the modern population. This shows that the benefits outweigh the legal and ethical concerns, in scientific studies targeting the young populations.

In summary, cardiovascular disease is considered as main factor causing premature deaths in industrialized countries. These patterns are also replicated in the UK population where most premature deaths are linked to CVD. CVD is a collection of various disease with common risk factors and linked to the stiffening of the artery walls. Among these conditions are the coronary heart disease, which is the most common form of CVD. CHD occurs due to atherosclerosis, which causes the artery networks found in the heart to reduce the blood supply. This leads to life-threatening complications, which when not addressed on time lead to premature deaths. Numerous risk factors lead to CHD, among them include genetic factors and lifestyle-related conditions. The marginalized communities, as exemplified by the South Asian population living in the UK have a higher risk of CHD. Consequently, this study recommends the promotion of cultural awareness in attempts to reduce care disparities affecting the South Asian communities. As a secondary CHD incidence prevention and management, UK healthcare system should enhance the management of various conditions such as lipid abnormalities, diabetes, obesity, hypertension, and cholesterol levels. This can be achieved by promoting the level of awareness. Based on the health belief model, this should facilitate behaviour management. Lastly, scientific evidence should also be enhanced to improve the evidence indicating the impacts of lifestyle and behaviour management in young populations.

References

**Primary Sources**

Bhatnagar, P., Wickramasinghe, K., Wilkins, E. and Townsend, N., 2016. Trends in the epidemiology of cardiovascular disease in the UK. *Heart*, pp.heartjnl-2016.

Danese, M.D., Gleeson, M., Kutikova, L., Griffiths, R.I., Azough, A., Khunti, K., Seshasai, S.R.K. and Ray, K.K., 2016. Estimating the economic burden of cardiovascular events in patients receiving lipid-modifying therapy in the UK. *BMJ open*, 6(8), p.e011805.

De Backer, G., Ambrosioni, E., Borch-Johnsen, K., Brotons, C., Cifkova, R., Dallongeville, J., Ebrahim, S., Faergeman, O., Graham, I., Mancia, G. and Cats, V.M., 2013. European guidelines on cardiovascular disease prevention in clinical practice: third joint task force of European and other societies on cardiovascular disease prevention in clinical practice (constituted by representatives of eight societies and by invited experts). *European heart journal*, 24(17), pp.1601-1610.

Hollis, B., Newson, R., Su, B., Onida, S., Davies, A., Ray, K., Tzoulaki, I. and Soljak, M., 2017. Coronary heart disease prevalence model for small populations. *Risk*, 3, p.4.

King, W., Lacey, A., White, J., Farewell, D., Dunstan, F. and Fone, D., 2017. Equity in healthcare for coronary heart disease, Wales (UK) 2004–2010: A population-based electronic cohort study. *PloS one*, 12(3), p.e0172618.

Williams, E.D., Nazroo, J.Y., Kooner, J.S. and Steptoe, A., 2010. Subgroup differences in psychosocial factors relating to coronary heart disease in the UK South Asian population. *Journal of psychosomatic research*, 69(4), pp.379-387.

Bhatnagar, P., Wickramasinghe, K., Wilkins, E. and Townsend, N., 2016. Trends in the epidemiology of cardiovascular disease in the UK. *Heart*, pp.heartjnl-2016.

Danese, M.D., Gleeson, M., Kutikova, L., Griffiths, R.I., Azough, A., Khunti, K., Seshasai, S.R.K. and Ray, K.K., 2016. Estimating the economic burden of cardiovascular events in patients receiving lipid-modifying therapy in the UK. *BMJ open*, 6(8), p.e011805.

De Backer, G., Ambrosioni, E., Borch-Johnsen, K., Brotons, C., Cifkova, R., Dallongeville, J., Ebrahim, S., Faergeman, O., Graham, I., Mancia, G. and Cats, V.M., 2013. European guidelines on cardiovascular disease prevention in clinical practice: third joint task force of European and other societies on cardiovascular disease prevention in clinical practice (constituted by representatives of eight societies and by invited experts). *European heart journal*, 24(17), pp.1601-1610.

Daoud, A., Jarmolych, J., Zumbo, A. And Florentin, R., 2014. Serum-cholesterol, diet, and coronary heart-disease in Africans and Asians in Uganda. *Science*, 344(6190), pp.1346-1348.

Hollis, B., Newson, R., Su, B., Onida, S., Davies, A., Ray, K., Tzoulaki, I. and Soljak, M., 2017. Coronary heart disease prevalence model for small populations. *Risk*, 3, p.4.

King, W., Lacey, A., White, J., Farewell, D., Dunstan, F. and Fone, D., 2017. Equity in healthcare for coronary heart disease, Wales (UK) 2004–2010: A population-based electronic cohort study. *PloS one*, 12(3), p.e0172618.

Osborn, D.P., Hardoon, S., Omar, R.Z., Holt, R.I., King, M., Larsen, J., Marston, L., Morris, R.W., Nazareth, I., Walters, K. and Petersen, I., 2015. Cardiovascular risk prediction models for people with severe mental illness: results from the prediction and management of cardiovascular risk in people with severe mental illnesses (PRIMROSE) research program. *JAMA psychiatry*, 72(2), pp.143-151.

Prince, M.J., Wu, F., Guo, Y., Robledo, L.M.G., O'Donnell, M., Sullivan, R. and Yusuf, S., 2015. The burden of disease in older people and implications for health policy and practice. *The Lancet*, 385(9967), pp.549-562.

Roth, G.A., Forouzanfar, M.H., Moran, A.E., Barber, R., Nguyen, G., Feigin, V.L., Naghavi, M., Mensah, G.A. and Murray, C.J., 2015. Demographic and epidemiologic drivers of global cardiovascular mortality. *New England Journal of Medicine*, 372(14), pp.1333-1341.

Tillin, T., Hughes, A.D., Whincup, P., Mayet, J., Sattar, N., McKeigue, P.M., Chaturvedi, N. and SABRE Study Group, 2014. Ethnicity and prediction of cardiovascular disease: performance of QRISK2 and Framingham scores in a UK tri-ethnic prospective cohort study (SABRE—Southall And Brent REvisited). *Heart*, *100*(1), pp.60-67.

Yusuf, S., Bosch, J., Dagenais, G., Zhu, J., Xavier, D., Liu, L., Pais, P., López-Jaramillo, P., Leiter, L.A., Dans, A. and Avezum, A., 2016. Cholesterol lowering in intermediate-risk persons without cardiovascular disease. *New England Journal of Medicine*, *374*(21), pp.2021-2031.

Williams, E.D., Nazroo, J.Y., Kooner, J.S. and Steptoe, A., 2010. Subgroup differences in psychosocial factors relating to coronary heart disease in the UK South Asian population. *Journal of psychosomatic research*, *69*(4), pp.379-387.

# YOUR KNOWLEDGE HAS VALUE

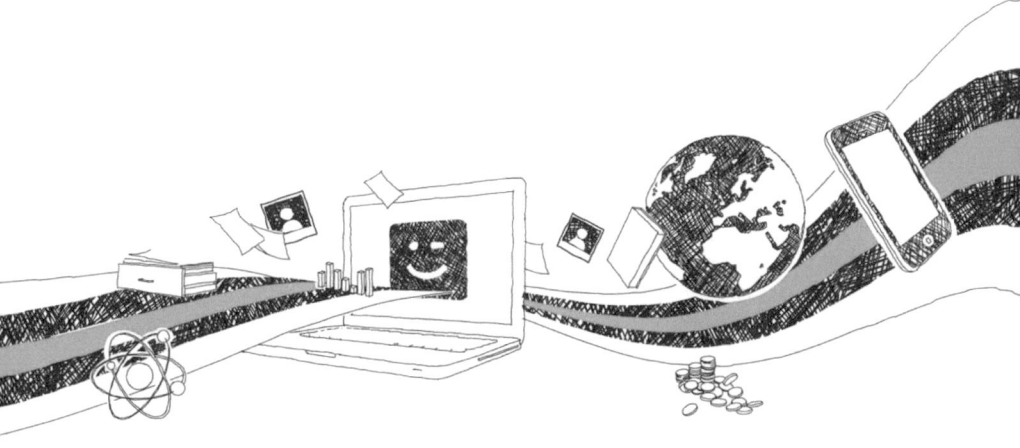

- We will publish your bachelor's and master's thesis, essays and papers

- Your own eBook and book - sold worldwide in all relevant shops

- Earn money with each sale

Upload your text at www.GRIN.com
and publish for free

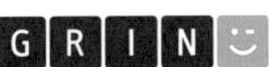